Mastering Your Fertility

A Step-by-Step Guide to Natural Birth Control and Pregnancy Achievement

Harmony Royce

DEDICATION

To individuals who want to accept and comprehend their fertility,

I hope this book helps you on your path to self-determination, education, and achieving your reproductive goals.

This work is dedicated to the loving, strong, and understanding families that motivate us to prioritize our reproductive health, as well as the committed healthcare professionals who support them.

I hope that the information in these pages will give you strength, encouragement, and hope as you travel your own road.

DISCLAIMER

This book contains information that should only be used for educational and informational reasons; it is not meant to be used as medical advice. Even though every attempt has been taken to guarantee the content's correctness and dependability, you should always seek the advice of a licensed healthcare provider before making any decisions pertaining to your family planning, fertility, or reproductive health.

Any negative effects or repercussions arising from the use or application of the information included in this book are not covered by the author or publisher. Individual experiences and outcomes may differ, and this material is not meant to replace tailored medical advice.

It is recommended that readers seek professional advice pertaining to their own health requirements and circumstances.

CONTENTS

ACKNOWLEDGMENTS

I want to express my sincere appreciation to everyone who helped make this book possible. I want to start by expressing my gratitude to my family and friends for their continuous support, understanding, and encouragement along this journey. Your support of my vision has always given me motivation.

I owe a debt of gratitude to the physicians, reproductive specialists, and educators whose wisdom and knowledge have influenced the information on these pages. Numerous people, including myself, have been inspired by your commitment to enhancing reproductive health.

We really appreciate the readers who are looking to learn more about fertility and feel more empowered about it. The significance of our work is driven by your willingness to investigate and comprehend your bodies.

I would also like to thank the many people and families who have so kindly shared their experiences and stories. Your voices give this book life and serve as a reminder of our common knowledge of fertility.

Finally, thank you for being change agents to everyone who works to raise public awareness and educate others about reproductive health. We can build an informed and capable community by working together.

CHAPTER 1

COMPREHENDING YOUR HEALTH IN REPRODUCTION

For women in particular, whose reproductive systems and hormonal balance play a crucial role in their physical, emotional, and mental health, reproductive health is fundamental to overall well-being. This chapter will offer a thorough examination of the female reproductive system, the hormones that control its operations, frequent problems with reproductive health that may occur, and how these disorders may impact fertility. It's important to know your reproductive health not only for family planning but also for general health maintenance and early detection of potential problems.

1.1 The Reproductive System of Females

The intricate network of organs and tissues that make up the female reproductive system is intended to generate eggs (ova), aid in fertilization, and support the growth of a fetus throughout pregnancy. We will examine the main elements of this system and their purposes in this section.

- **Ovaries:** On either side of the uterus are two tiny, almond-shaped organs known as the ovaries. Their main jobs are to release vital hormones like progesterone and estrogen and to produce eggs. During the reproductive years of a woman, the ovaries release a mature egg once a month through a process known as ovulation.

- **Fallopian Tubes:** The ovaries and uterus are connected by these tiny tubes. An egg released by an ovary passes via the fallopian tube and may fertilize when it comes into contact with sperm. The fallopian tubes are vital in the early stages of pregnancy because they act as the egg's route.

- **Uterus:** During pregnancy, the uterus, sometimes referred to as the womb, is a pear-shaped, muscular organ that houses and feeds a growing fetus. Every month, the endometrium, or lining of the uterus, thickens in anticipation of a fertilized egg. During menstruation, the lining sheds if fertilization is unsuccessful.

- **Cervix:** The narrow, lower portion of the uterus that joins the vagina is called the cervix. It opens during birthing to facilitate the baby's passage and permits menstrual blood to exit the uterus.

Menstruation and Cycle:

One important determinant of a woman's reproductive health is her menstrual cycle. Although it can vary from person to person, it usually lasts 28 days. There are four primary phases to it:

1. Menstrual Phase: The uterine lining sheds at the beginning of the cycle, causing menstrual bleeding.

2. Follicular Phase: Ovulation marks the end of this phase, which starts on the first day of menstruation. Follicle-stimulating hormone (FSH), which is released by the pituitary gland during this period, causes the ovaries to form follicles containing immature eggs.

3. Ovulation: A mature egg is released from one of the ovaries midway through the cycle due to an increase in luteinizing hormone (LH). This window is fertile.

4. Luteal Phase: The corpus luteum, which is formed by the ruptured follicle after ovulation, secretes progesterone to prime the uterus for a possible pregnancy. Menstruation results from the corpus luteum disintegrating if the egg is not fertilized.

Why It's Important to Know Reproductive Health:

Gaining and maintaining a natural pregnancy requires a thorough understanding of menstrual cycles and reproductive anatomy. In addition to using this information for family planning, women can track ovulation to identify viable windows and identify any abnormalities that might point to health issues. Furthermore, by being aware of the hormonal cues provided by the menstrual cycle, women can detect irregularities in their cycles and take early action to address any potential risks to their reproductive health.

1.2 Women's Hormonal Regulation

A key factor in controlling the female reproductive system is hormones. They maintain reproductive health, facilitate the menstrual cycle, and get the body ready for conception. We'll go over each of the main hormones involved and their functions in detail here.

- **Estrogen:** Mainly produced by the ovaries, this is one of the key sex hormones for women. Estrogen plays a critical role in the development of secondary sexual features (hips and breasts), menstrual cycle regulation, and reproductive tissue health. Estrogen levels rise throughout the first half of the menstrual cycle, which causes the endometrial lining to thicken in anticipation of a possible pregnancy.

- **Progesterone:** The ovaries release progesterone following ovulation, which combines with estrogen to ready the uterus for a fertilized egg. Progesterone supports uterine lining maintenance in the event of pregnancy. Menstruation is brought on by a decline in progesterone levels in the absence of pregnancy.

- **Follicle-stimulating hormone (FSH) and luteinizing hormone (LH)**: LH and FSH, which are produced by the pituitary gland, control how the ovaries operate. During the follicular phase, FSH promotes the development of ovarian follicles, and a spike in LH causes ovulation, which releases the egg from the follicle.

Changes in Hormones and Their Effect on Fertility:

Fertility is determined by the complex interactions between hormones during the menstrual cycle. A healthy menstrual cycle and ovulation depend on the proper ratio of progesterone to estrogen. Anovulation, or the absence of ovulation, and luteal phase abnormalities are two disorders that can result from imbalances in these hormones and impair a woman's ability to become pregnant. Tracking these hormones can reveal information about the status of fertility and aid in the diagnosis of underlying problems linked to hormone imbalances.

1.3 Typical Problems with Reproductive Health

Women frequently have a number of reproductive health problems that might make it difficult for them to become pregnant, keep their menstrual cycle regular, or cause excruciating pain. In order to manage these diseases and maintain fertility, early detection and treatment are essential. Below are some of the most prevalent reproductive health conditions:

- **Endometriosis:** This disorder is brought on by tissue that grows outside of the uterus, usually on the ovaries, fallopian tubes, or pelvic lining, and resembles the endometrium. Because endometriosis causes inflammation and scar tissue to build in the reproductive organs, it can lead to painful periods, ongoing pelvic pain, and problems with conception.

- **Symptoms:** Severe menstrual cramps, profuse bleeding, pain during sex, and trouble getting pregnant.

- **Diagnosis:** Pelvic exams, ultrasounds, and laparoscopies a minor surgical procedure can all be used to detect endometriosis.

- **Treatment Options**: In order to treat endometrial tissue growth, hormonal therapy may be used, as well as surgery to remove extra tissue. Pain management is one option. Fertility therapies such as in vitro fertilization (IVF) could be required in extreme circumstances.

- **Polycystic Ovary Syndrome (PCOS):** An excess of androgens (male hormones) and several little cysts on the ovaries are the hallmarks of this hormonal condition. It may result in weight gain, acne, irregular periods, and excessive hair growth. Because of inconsistent or absent ovulation, PCOS is one of the main reasons for infertility.

- **Symptoms:** Weight gain, acne, hirsutism (excessive hair growth), irregular or nonexistent periods.

- **Diagnosis:** Pelvic ultrasounds, blood tests to assess hormone levels, and symptom evaluation are commonly used in the diagnosis process.

- **Treatment Options:** If pregnancy is desired, treatment options include hormonal birth control to regulate periods, lifestyle modifications (such as weight loss and exercise), and drugs to encourage ovulation.

- **Ovarian Cysts:** These are sacs filled with fluid that grow on the ovaries. Although the majority of ovarian cysts are benign and disappear on their own, some can hurt, bloat, or interfere with fertility especially if they burst or get very large.

- **Symptoms:** irregular menstrual periods, bloating, pain during sex, and pelvic pain.

- **Diagnosis:** Pelvic examinations or ultrasounds are typically used to identify ovarian cysts.

- **Treatment Options:** Ovarian cysts usually go away on their own. Larger or more chronic cysts, however, could need to be surgically removed or treated with hormones.

How These Conditions Affect Fertility:

Endometriosis, PCOS, and ovarian cysts are just a few of the conditions that can significantly affect a woman's ability to conceive by interfering with ovulation, causing obstructions in the reproductive canal, or changing hormone levels. Women should visit a doctor if they have symptoms like irregular periods, excruciating menstrual pain, or trouble getting pregnant. Maintaining fertility and enhancing reproductive health depend heavily on the early detection and treatment of these disorders.

Gaining more control over your body, fertility, and overall well-being is possible when you are aware of your reproductive health. Knowing more about your reproductive system's workings and potential problems will help you make better decisions about family planning, medical treatments, and lifestyle choices that promote long-term reproductive health.

CHAPTER 2

FERTILITY AWARENESS METHOD (FAM) OVERVIEW

The natural, scientifically supported Fertility Awareness Method (FAM) helps women understand their menstrual cycles in order to either become pregnant or avoid getting pregnant. FAM is a potent family planning tool because it enables women to track their fertility in real time by getting attentive to the body's signals. This chapter will cover the basics of FAM, how to determine the viable window, and methods for tracking fertility signals on a daily basis.

2.1 Fundamentals of Awareness of Fertility

Using the Fertility Awareness Method (FAM), a natural family planning technique, a woman can track her menstrual cycle to identify her fertile and infertile days. It is predicated on the observation and interpretation of biological cues that signal ovulation, the critical process that releases a mature egg from the ovary in order to facilitate conception.

History and Definition of FAM:

The scientific understanding of reproductive physiology, in particular the time of ovulation during the menstrual cycle, is the basis of family anthropology. Although it has been used in various forms for millennia, it only received formal recognition in the 20th century due to advancements in reproductive health. The current FAM system was created to give women a natural method of preventing and obtaining conception, as well as an alternative to hormonal contraception. It necessitates regular observation of the cervix's position, basal body temperature, and cervical mucus physical indicators of fertility.

How to Use FAM to Achieve Pregnancy and Natural Birth Control:

By determining the fertile window and refraining from unprotected sexual activity during this period, or by employing barrier techniques like condoms, FAM can be utilized to prevent pregnancy. To increase their chances of conceiving, couples who are attempting to get pregnant might utilize FAM to schedule their sexual activity during the most fertile times of the month. Accurately analyzing fertility cues to anticipate ovulation is essential for both applications.

1. **For Natural Birth Control:** During the fertile window, couples utilizing FAM to prevent conception refrain from sexual activity or use non-hormonal contraception. With a normal use failure rate of about 2–5%, FAM can be just as successful as hormonal contraceptives when used consistently and precisely.

2. **For Pregnancy Achievement:** Those who are trying to conceive can determine when they are most fertile, which is usually the day of ovulation and the few days before, and take sexual activity throughout this window.

Comparing FAM to Other Natural Family Planning Methods: Although FAM is sometimes included in the same category as other natural family planning (NFP) techniques, it's crucial to set it apart from other strategies:

1. **The Rhythm Method:** This more traditional

approach uses calendar computations predicated on the idea that ovulation happens on day 14. However, because women's cycles vary widely, the rhythm technique is less accurate and successful compared to FAM, which evaluates genuine biological indicators rather than depending on average cycle durations.

2. **Sympto-Thermal Method:** This is a more sophisticated version of FAM that involves tracking cervical mucus, basal body temperature, and occasionally other physical symptoms like breast soreness or pain during the menstrual cycle.

3. **Billings Ovulation Method:** This approach, which may be less precise, just monitors cervical mucus; it does not check cervical position or temperature.

2.2 Fertile Window Understanding

The foundation of FAM is an understanding of the fruitful window. The time during the menstrual cycle when pregnancy is most likely to occur is referred to as the fertile window. Since sperm can survive in the female reproductive system for up to five days and eggs can remain viable for 12 to 24 hours after ovulation, this usually takes place over the course of six days, including the day of ovulation and the five days before it.

Ovulation and Fertility: Determining the Cycle's Most Fertile Days:

A developed egg is discharged from the ovary into the fallopian tube during ovulation so that sperm can fertilize it. Because the egg is ready for fertilization on the day of ovulation and the two days preceding it, these are typically the most fertile times. Recognizing these days is important for conception as well as natural contraception. By keeping an eye out for particular reproductive indicators, FAM offers the means to identify this window.

Differences in Basal Body Temperature and Cervical Mucus:

Two of the most dependable indicators of fertility during the menstrual cycle are variations in basal body temperature (BBT) and cervical mucus:

- **Cervical Mucus:** The quantity and consistency of cervical mucus vary during the menstrual cycle.

Right after menstruation, the mucus is usually mild and dry. As ovulation approaches, estrogen levels rise, causing the mucus to become more plentiful, slick, and stretchy similar to raw egg whites. This kind of mucus indicates peak fertility and is ideal for sperm motility and survival.

- **Basal Body Temperature (BBT)**: After waking up and before engaging in any activity, a woman's BBT is her body's lowest resting temperature. Progesterone raises body temperature (BBT) after ovulation, usually by 0.5 to 1 degree Fahrenheit. Although this rise is a retrospective signal that is, it indicates that ovulation has already taken place rather than indicating when it will it can be used to confirm that ovulation has occurred.

Using Your Cycle Chart to Precisely Predict Ovulation:
Recording daily observations of BBT and cervical mucus on a fertility chart or with a digital fertility tracker is the process of charting your cycle. Over time, trends will emerge, allowing you to forecast ovulation and determine the viable window more accurately. Many women find it

beneficial to utilize a mix of FAM indicators—mucus, temperature, and cervical position—to improve accuracy.

Actionable Charting Tips

1. Take your basal body temperature each morning at the same time before you get out of bed.

2. Keep an eye on and record the amount and consistency of cervical mucus during the day.

3. It is optional to verify your reproductive status further by examining your cervical position, which is covered below.

4. Look for trends in the chart and make use of the data from prior months to predict when the next cycle will be fruitful.

2.3 Methods of Daily Monitoring

Maintaining a good FAM practice requires daily monitoring. Women can confidently determine whether they are fertile and infertile by monitoring bodily indicators of fertility on a daily basis. FAM becomes more dependable the more regularly and precisely these indicators are observed.

Using a Basal Body Thermometer: A basal body thermometer measures temperature to two decimal places (e.g., 98.26°F), making it more sensitive than a standard thermometer. This level of accuracy is required to identify the minute rise in body temperature that follows ovulation.

How to Use:

1. Take your temperature at the same time each morning, preferably following three hours of sound sleep.

2. To guarantee consistent readings, use the same thermometer and technique (rectally, vaginally, or orally) every day.

3. Quickly note the temperature on a fertility tracking chart or smartphone app.

4. After ovulation, watch for the slight increase in BBT; this shift usually indicates the end of the viable window.

Aware of the Importance of Fluid and Cervical Position:

Throughout the menstrual cycle, the cervix experiences

minor alterations in addition to changes in mucus. The cervix gets softer, higher, more open, and wetter around ovulation to facilitate sperm passage.

How to Check Cervical Position:

1. Cleanse your hands, then feel the cervix with your fingers inserted softly into the vagina.

2. The cervix will feel softer (like the lips) and be higher, making it more difficult to reach, on fertile days. Additionally, the cervix opens up somewhat.

3. The cervix returns to its lower, firmer, closed posture following ovulation, which aids in preventing bacteria or sperm from entering the uterus.

Monitoring Affective and Physical Shifts as Signs of Fertility:

During their reproductive window, some women experience extra physical and emotional changes, such as:

1. "Mittelschmerz" is a term for mild abdominal cramps or breast soreness.

2. An increase in libido or vitality around ovulation.

3. Modest mood swings, an enhanced sense of smell, or other minor adjustments.

While each woman may experience these symptoms differently, when combined with other FAM signs, they might offer additional information to validate the fertile window.

The Fertility Awareness Method is an effective, all-natural strategy for controlling fertility, regardless of whether getting pregnant is the aim or not. Women can obtain important knowledge about their reproductive health by employing daily monitoring tools, recognizing the viable window, and comprehending the fundamentals of the menstrual cycle. As with any technique, accuracy and consistency are key to success, and the more a woman pays attention to her body's reproductive cues, the more successful FAM becomes.

CHAPTER 3

NATURAL FERTILIZATION

There's more to naturally becoming pregnant than simply scheduling sex around ovulation. It necessitates an all-encompassing strategy that takes both couples' health and wellbeing into account. Couples can greatly increase their chances of getting pregnant by making the most of their lifestyle, mental, and physical components. This chapter will cover the essentials of priming the body for conception, maximizing male fecundity, and knowing how to make the process of attempting to conceive through sex that enhances fertility even more enjoyable.

3.1 Getting Your Body Ready for Fertility

It's important to get your body ready for pregnancy before trying to get pregnant. To increase the likelihood of conception and a successful pregnancy, this entails establishing an environment in which both the egg and the sperm may flourish.

Dietary Guidelines and Supplements to Enhance Fertility:

Fertility is fundamentally influenced by nutrition. Eating a well-balanced diet full of vital nutrients supports both good reproductive function and general wellness. Important nutrients for sperm production consist of:

1. **Folic Acid:** Vital for reproductive health, folic acid is also known to prevent neural tube abnormalities. A minimum of 400–600 micrograms of folic acid should be consumed by women who are attempting to get pregnant each day, either through food or supplements.

2. **Iron:** Iron contributes to the development of healthy blood, which is necessary to sustain pregnancy. Low iron levels in women may make it harder for them to get pregnant. Good sources of iron include foods like beans, lean meats, and leafy greens.

3. **Omega-3 Fatty Acids:** Omega-3s enhance hormone production and improve blood flow to reproductive organs. Nuts like walnuts, flaxseeds, and fatty fish,

as well as fish oil supplements, can improve fertility.

4. **Zinc:** A vital mineral for sperm health, ovulation, and hormone production, zinc affects both male and female fertility. Nuts, seeds, and shellfish all contain it.

In addition to a nutrient-rich diet, several supplements can further increase fertility, particularly if nutrient levels are low:

1. **Coenzyme Q10:** Known to increase egg quality, especially in women over 35.

2. **Vitamin D:** Supplementation may be required, particularly for people with limited sun exposure, as low levels of this vitamin have been related to decreased fertility.

3. **Prenatal Vitamins:** Prenatal vitamins can supply the essential vitamins and minerals required for pregnancy even before fertilization.

Modifications to Lifestyle: Physical Activity, Stress Reduction, and Detoxification:

- **Workout:** Hormonal balance and circulation are enhanced by regular, moderate exercise, both of which are essential for reproductive health. Excessive or severe activity, on the other hand, may have the opposite impact, lowering fertility and upsetting menstrual cycles. Maintaining an active lifestyle without going overboard is the aim. Walking, yoga, and swimming are great exercises to support fertility.

- **Stress Management:** By interfering with hormone levels and ovulation, long-term stress can have a deleterious effect on fertility. Stress levels can be managed with the use of stress reduction practices including mindfulness, meditation, yoga, or even acupuncture. Relaxing yourself and getting enough sleep (7-9 hours per night) are essential for maintaining reproductive health and managing stress.

- **Detoxification:** Processed foods, home chemicals, and environmental toxins can build up in the body and disrupt hormone balance and fertility. The body can be cleansed of toxic substances by gently detoxifying, which includes cutting out processed foods, alcohol, and caffeine and concentrating on natural, organic foods. Hormonal health can also be enhanced by making sure that your surroundings are free of endocrine disruptors, which are present in some plastics, cosmetics, and cleaning supplies.

Age and General Health's Effect on Fertility:

One of the most important factors influencing fertility, especially for women, is age. A woman's egg supply is limited from birth, and as she ages, her egg quality and quantity decrease. The highest fertility rates are usually found in women under 35; however, chances of getting pregnant naturally decline dramatically beyond the age of 40. Men stay fertile for longer, but as they age, the quality of their sperm also deteriorates. For both couples, maintaining good general health through frequent check-ups, healthy diet, and lifestyle management is vital for maximizing fertility.

3.2 Improving Fertility in Men

Since the condition of the sperm directly impacts the chance of successful fertilization, male fertility is equally vital to conception. It's important to pay attention to lifestyle choices and health issues that can affect sperm motility, viability, and production in order to maximize sperm quality.

The Function of Health and Sperm Quality in Conception:

Three primary factors:

1. count
2. motility
3. morphology

These determine the health of sperm.

- **Count** denotes the quantity of sperm in a specific sample of semen. The probability of one sperm reaching and fertilizing the egg rises with the number of sperm.
- **Motility** is the measure of sperm motility. For the sperm to reach the egg in the fallopian tube, they must swim effectively. Reduced motility lowers the likelihood of conceiving.
- **Morphology** describes the sperm's form. Typically, healthy sperm have an oval head and a lengthy tail. Sperm with unusual shapes could have trouble

breaking through the egg.

Lifestyle Factors Affecting Viability and Sperm Production:

A number of lifestyle decisions can influence sperm production and total fertility in a favorable or negative way:

- **Diet and Nutrition:** A healthy diet is essential for male fertility, just as it is for female fertility. Fruits, vegetables, nuts, and seeds are high in antioxidants and can shield sperm from oxidative stress. Vitamin C, zinc, and selenium are especially helpful in raising the caliber of sperm.

- **Avoiding Toxins:** Sperm quality can be considerably lowered by exposure to toxins, such as smoking, binge drinking, using recreational drugs, and exposure to environmental contaminants. Men who want to increase their fertility should abstain from smoke, drink in moderation, and minimize their exposure to dangerous chemicals.

- **Heat Exposure:** The testicles are situated outside of the main body cavity because sperm production prefers slightly colder temperatures than those of the rest of the body. Prolonged exposure to heat—such as from hot tubs, saunas, or tight clothing—can affect sperm production.

Measuring and Enhancing Sperm Morphology, Count, and Motility:

Semen analysis is frequently the first step in assessing male fertility for couples who are having trouble conceiving. Sperm count, motility, and morphology are evaluated by this test. If sperm quality is not at its best, the following interventions can be helpful:

- **Supplements:** It has been shown that certain supplements, such as folic acid, L-carnitine, and Coenzyme Q10, can improve sperm health. Antioxidants such as vitamin C and E, together with omega-3 fatty acids, also enhance sperm motility and quality.

- **Lifestyle Modifications**: Reducing alcohol use,

controlling stress, giving up smoking, and keeping a healthy weight are all factors that improve sperm quality.

- **Regular Exercise:** Regularly doing moderate-intensity physical activity increases testosterone levels and enhances motility and sperm count. Excessive activity, on the other hand, especially sitting-intensive exercises like cycling, can have a deleterious effect on sperm production.

3.3 Fertility-Boosting Intercourse

A healthy, deep relationship and the appropriate timing of sexual activity are crucial elements of conception. In order to increase the likelihood of conception, fertility-enhancing sex focuses on maximizing the emotional, technical, and temporal aspects of sexual activity.

- **Scheduling Sexual Activity for Conception:** A woman is most fertile during her ovulation window, which usually happens around the middle of her menstrual cycle. Because the egg only survives for

12 to 24 hours after being released from the female reproductive system, while sperm can stay in the system for up to five days, the five days preceding and following ovulation are the most crucial for conception.

- During this fertile window, couples should have sex every one to two days to increase the likelihood of becoming pregnant. Regular sexual activity is not required and may potentially be detrimental if the male partner has low sperm counts because it lowers sperm concentration. Having sex every other day promotes a greater sperm concentration in each ejaculation.

- Ovulation predictor kits (OPKs) or fertility tracking applications can assist couples in pinpointing the exact moment of ovulation, guaranteeing that sexual activity occurs during the most fertile time.

- **Optimal Sexual Positions for Sperm Transport:** Although no research has conclusively shown that any particular sexual position increases the likelihood of conception, it is believed that positions that permit deeper penetration, like missionary or rear-entry, encourage the deposition of sperm closer to the cervix. This could make it more likely for sperm to get to the egg.

Certain specialists advise the lady to lie down for ten to fifteen minutes after the sexual encounter in order to increase the chances of the sperm entering the fallopian tubes. While gravity plays a very small part in conception, this procedure might have a small benefit for sperm movement.

Preserving Closeness Throughout the Fertilization Process:

The relationship between a couple may occasionally suffer as a result of the emotional strain of trying to conceive. Encouraging emotional intimacy and connection throughout the process is crucial. Relishing the moment instead of seeing sex as a method to conceive. This will release tension. Having an open line of communication, doing relaxation exercises together, and making sure that each spouse feels emotionally supported are all essential to keeping the relationship strong throughout this period.

Maintaining physical and mental well-being is essential to getting pregnant naturally. The likelihood of conception can be greatly increased by optimizing male fertility, timing fertility-enhancing sex, and preparing the body through appropriate nutrition, lifestyle changes, and stress management. Couples can collaborate to create the best environment for conception and a safe pregnancy by acknowledging and honoring the body's natural cycles and requirements.

CHAPTER 4

NATURAL PREGNANCY PREVENTION

Naturally avoiding pregnancy is a deliberate decision that calls for meticulous preparation, consistency, and a thorough awareness of the body's reproductive cues. The Fertility Awareness Method (FAM), in particular, and other natural methods of contraception will be discussed in this chapter along with their underlying principles. Along with highlighting non-hormonal alternatives, it will provide advice on how to use birth control for various life stages and medical conditions.

4.1 Comprehending Your Contraceptive Cycle

Tracking physiological indicators helps natural family planning approaches like FAM identify fertile and infertile times in the menstrual cycle. When utilized appropriately, FAM can be a useful method of preventing pregnancy when combined with other forms of contraception or abstinence from sexual activity during fertile periods.

The FAM Factor That Explains Its Use in Pregnancy Prevention:

The Fertility Awareness Method is built in a detailed understanding of a woman's reproductive cycle. Hormonal variations that control ovulation and menstruation define the periods of fertility and infertility that occur with each menstrual cycle. With the aid of FAM, women can determine when their fertile window is, which usually falls around ovulation, and utilize other forms of contraception or refrain from sexual activity at that time.

The technique monitors and records important signs of fertility, like:

1. **Basal Body Temperature (BBT):** A woman's body temperature increases somewhat following ovulation as a result of an increase in progesterone. Time of day temperatures over several cycles can be used to determine when ovulation occurs.

2. **Cervical Mucus:** High fertility is indicated by cervical mucus that is more plentiful, stretchy, and slippery as ovulation draws near. It resembles raw

egg whites. It is crucial to track mucus changes in order to determine the fertile window.

3. **Cervical Position:** The cervix becomes soft, high, and open during the fertile window and firmer and lower outside of it. This may serve as an additional marker of fertility for women who are aware of their own menstrual cycles.

FAM can be as effective as 98% of the time when used appropriately and consistently, but this needs a thorough understanding of one's physiology and rigorous adherence to tracking procedures. An unplanned pregnancy might result from errors in charting, misreading indications, or having sex during fertile days.

Identifying Ovulation Symptoms to Prevent Fertile Times:

Ovulation, the most fertile time in a woman's cycle, is defined as the release of an egg from the ovary. When utilizing natural approaches to avoid pregnancy, the key is understanding the indications of ovulation. In addition to BBT and cervical mucus alterations, other symptoms could be:

1. **Mittelschmerz:** Around the time of ovulation, some women have moderate abdominal cramps or soreness on one side.

2. **Increased Libido:** Due to hormonal changes during ovulation, many women report having a stronger desire for sex.

3. **Breast Tenderness:** Some women experience breast tenderness or sensitivity during ovulation.

Couples can successfully avoid pregnancy by recognizing these symptoms, abstaining from sexual activity, or utilizing barrier techniques throughout the fertile window.

Monitoring Non-Regular Cycles and Modifying FAM Consequently:

FAM can still be used by women with irregular cycles, but it could need more effort on their part. Irregular cycles may be influenced by causes such as stress, sickness, or hormone abnormalities. It is important to regularly monitor several fertility indicators since women with disorders like polycystic ovarian syndrome (PCOS) or those approaching perimenopause may have irregular ovulation. In these circumstances:

1. More accurate information on fertility can be obtained by **cross-referencing multiple fertility indicators**, such as BBT, cervical mucus, and cervical position.

2. **Adapting methods for variable cycles:** To better tailor FAM to their particular circumstances, women with irregular cycles may find it helpful to speak with a healthcare professional skilled in natural family planning.

4.2 Other Natural Contraceptive Options

While FAM is a well-liked option for people looking for natural contraception, there are other non-hormonal options that can be used in addition to or instead of hormones to prevent pregnancy. These techniques are adaptable and might be simpler for some people to implement in their everyday lives.

Introduction to Barrier Methods:

Cervical Caps, Diaphragms, and Condoms: Barrier techniques work by physically preventing sperm from attaching itself to the egg. Among these techniques are:

1. **Condoms:** Among the most popular barrier techniques are male and female condoms. They also provide the extra advantage of STI (sexually transmitted infection) prevention. When used properly, condom effectiveness ranges from 85 to 98 percent.

2. **Diaphragms:** To cover the cervix and keep sperm from accessing the uterus, a diaphragm is a shallow, flexible cup that is placed into the vagina. For best results, diaphragms should be worn in conjunction with spermicide and kept in place for a minimum of six hours following sexual activity. Their efficacy ranges between 88-94%.

3. **Cervical Caps:** Cervical caps fit over the cervix more snugly and are smaller than diaphragms. They also need spermicide and, depending on whether a woman has given birth before, have an efficacy rate of roughly 71–86%.

For women who wish to avoid the negative consequences of hormonal techniques, barrier methods offer reversible, non-hormonal contraception.

Using Non-Hormonal IUDs with Spermicide:

1. **Spermicides**: These are chemical agents that, before reaching the egg, paralyze or destroy sperm. Spermicides can be used alone or in conjunction with barrier techniques and come in a variety of forms, including gels, creams, foams, and suppositories. Spermicide by itself, however, is only 71-28% effective; it works best when combined with other strategies.

2. **IUDs Without Hormones:** The copper intrauterine device (IUD) is a long-term contraceptive method that is very successful in keeping sperm in a hazardous environment. Because copper alters sperm motility, fertilization cannot occur. With an over 99% success rate, the non-hormonal copper IUD has a 10- to 12-year lifespan. For women looking for a long-term, low-maintenance, natural form of birth control, it is a good choice.

Evaluating Natural Therapies Against Hormonal Contraceptives:

When applied properly, natural methods can be very effective, but they need more work and dedication than hormonal approaches. When used properly, hormonal contraceptives, like birth control tablets, patches, and intrauterine systems (IUS), have effectiveness rates that are often higher over 99%. But a majority of women would rather use natural ways to avoid hormonal side effects like mood swings, weight gain, and increased risk of blood clots. The decision between hormonal and natural techniques ultimately comes down to personal taste, way of life, and health factors.

4.3 Managing Birth Control at Various Stages of Life

Women's preferences and needs for birth control frequently change as they go through different phases of life. Women's decisions to avoid getting pregnant naturally might be influenced by a variety of factors, including approaching menopause, medical issues, or stopping hormonal birth control.

Modifying Contraceptive Techniques During Menopause and Perimenopause:

The period that precedes menopause, known as perimenopause, is when fertility starts to decrease and menstrual periods may become erratic. Contraception is still necessary until menopause, which is defined as 12 consecutive months without a period is proven because women who are perimenopausal can still become pregnant.

- **FAM during Perimenopause:** Hormonal variations that alter the predictability of ovulation can make tracking fertility during perimenopause more difficult. To achieve effective contraception, women may need to use barrier techniques in addition to natural methods like FAM.

- **Non-hormonal IUDs and Barrier Techniques**: Women who experience more irregular cycles could find barrier techniques or copper IUDs more convenient because they don't rely on hormonal cycles to function. These techniques offer effective birth control without interfering with the body's normal hormonal cycles.

After menopause, birth control is no longer necessary, however some women may still prefer to utilize barrier techniques for protection against STIs, especially if they have new or multiple sexual partners.

Birth Control Considerations for Women with Medical illnesses (e.g., PCOS, Endometriosis): When selecting a birth control method, women with medical illnesses like polycystic ovarian syndrome (PCOS) or endometriosis may need to take additional variables into account.

1. **PCOS:** Women with PCOS frequently have inconsistent ovulation, which makes it more challenging to use FAM correctly. An increasingly dependable and constant method of contraception could be offered by copper IUDs or barrier techniques.

2. **Endometriosis:** Non-hormonal choices like diaphragms, condoms, or the copper IUD may be preferable for women with endometriosis who wish to avoid hormonal techniques. But since endometriosis symptoms are frequently treated with hormone medications, women should collaborate with their healthcare professionals to find a solution that balances symptom management with the requirement for contraception.

Changing from chemical Birth Control to FAM: It may take several months for a woman's menstrual cycle to stabilize after stopping chemical birth control. It may be challenging to interpret fertility signals during this period, therefore women adjusting to FAM should think about utilizing barrier techniques.

1. **Post-hormonal Cycle Regulation:** The body takes some time to return to its normal cycle after using hormonal birth control, which suppresses ovulation. If a woman wants to use FAM only for contraception, she should wait at least three months to check her fertility indicators.

2. **Using Barrier Methods During the Transition**: Condoms or a diaphragm might offer peace of mind and protection against pregnancy until cycles become more regular.

Naturally avoiding getting pregnant can be an effective solution for many women, but it necessitates a dedication to body awareness and ongoing education about available techniques. Women can choose from a variety of natural choices that suit their tastes and health concerns, including non-hormonal IUDs, barrier techniques, and free-form IUDs. Contraception options may need to be modified as life stages change, but natural techniques can offer empowering and successful family planning solutions with proper preparation.

CHAPTER 5

TECHNOLOGIES FOR ASSISTED REPRODUCTION (ART) ADVANCES

Millions of single people and couples who battle infertility now have hope thanks to assisted reproductive technologies (ART), which have completely changed the field of fertility. The options for conception using these techniques are limited, but they also grow with science and technology. This chapter explores the most popular ART techniques, new developments that have increased their efficacy, and the moral and economical ramifications of these treatments.

5.1 Overview of ART Processes

Assisted Reproductive Technologies refer to a range of medical procedures intended to assist people in becoming pregnant when naturally occurring conception is difficult or impossible. For those experiencing infertility for medical, anatomical, or unknown causes, these methods have emerged as an indispensable resource.

Recap of Typical ART Techniques: IUI, IVF, and ICSI:
While there are several techniques used in Assisted Reproductive Technology (ART), Intrauterine Insemination (IUI), In Vitro Fertilization (IVF), and Intracytoplasmic Sperm Injection (ICSI) are three of the most widely utilized techniques. The goals of each of these treatments vary based on the underlying cause of infertility.

1. **Intrauterine Insemination (IUI):** To increase the likelihood that sperm will reach and fertilize the egg, sperm is inserted directly into a woman's uterus during ovulation. When using donor sperm or for couples experiencing mild male factor infertility, IUI is frequently advised.

2. **In Vitro Fertilization (IVF):** One of the most popular ART techniques is IVF. It entails inducing the ovaries to release several eggs, extracting these eggs, fertilizing them in a laboratory with sperm, and then putting one or more embryos into the uterus. IVF is frequently used to treat a variety of infertility

problems, such as severe male infertility, advanced mother age, and obstructed fallopian tubes.

3. **The procedure known as Intracytoplasmic Sperm Injection (ICSI)** is a specific type of IVF that is mostly used to treat infertility in men. To aid in fertilization, a single sperm is delivered straight into an egg during this process. When there is poor sperm quality, such as low motility or aberrant morphology, it is very helpful.

For those who are having trouble becoming pregnant, these procedures provide a variety of options that can be tailored to the patient's particular situation and medical background.

ART's Place in the Treatment of Infertility:

The treatment of infertility, which affects 10–15% of couples globally, is greatly aided by ART. Male factor infertility, hormonal imbalances, age-related loss in fertility, and anatomical anomalies are some of the reasons for infertility. When less invasive surgeries or medication-based reproductive treatments don't work, ART sometimes becomes the only viable route to becoming a biological parent.

ART treatments, especially IVF and ICSI, are essential for resolving more complicated infertility situations. As an illustration:

1. **Ovulation Disorders:** IVF, in which ovulation is surgically induced and eggs are extracted straight from the ovaries, may be beneficial for women who either have irregular ovulation cycles or do not ovulate at all.

2. **Tubal Blockages or Damage:** IVF completely avoids the fallopian tubes, making it a feasible choice for women in situations when natural conception is not possible due to blocked or damaged tubes.

3. **Male Factor Infertility:** ICSI provides a remedy by injecting sperm directly into the egg in cases of severe male infertility where sperm count, motility, or morphology are affected.

ART has developed into a vital tool in contemporary reproductive medicine, giving individuals and couples who previously faced the possibility of childlessness hope and observable outcomes.

Achievement Rates and Influential Elements:

The age of the patient, the reason for the infertility, and the particular ART technique utilized are some of the variables that affect the success rates of ART procedures. For instance, women under the age of 35 have a much greater success rate with IVF (40–50%) than do those over 40 (10–20%).

The effectiveness of ART therapies is influenced by various factors:

1. **Age**: As a woman ages, her egg quality and quantity decrease, which reduces the efficacy of ART treatments for women over 35, especially those over 40.

2. **Embryo Quality**: An important factor in determining the effectiveness of ART is the health and viability of the embryos. Genetically defective embryos have a lower chance of implanting and developing into a viable pregnancy.

3. **Underlying Health Conditions:** Uterine abnormalities, endometriosis, and polycystic ovarian

syndrome (PCOS) can all have an impact on the prognosis for assisted reproductive technology (ART). It can help to treat these issues before beginning ART.

4. **Sperm Quality:** A number of parameters related to male fertility, including motility, morphology, and sperm count, are important in determining how well ICSI techniques work.

Although many people's success rates have increased thanks to ART, each situation is different and results might vary greatly. These rates are rising as a result of ongoing technological developments, providing promise for more reliable outcomes.

5.2 Advances in Reproductive Health Technology

New advancements in ART technology are making these operations more accessible and effective as they develop. New developments are opening up more options for individuals and couples who might not have had luck using conventional ART techniques.

The Most Recent Developments in Embryo Transfer and Egg Retrieval:

ART outcomes have been markedly improved by advancements in the techniques of egg retrieval and embryo transfer. Patient comfort, egg viability, and successful embryo implantation are given top priority in modern procedures.

1. **Egg Retrieval:** Better synchronization of egg development has been made possible by advancements in ovarian stimulation procedures, making egg retrieval more successful. These techniques increase the likelihood of obtaining high-quality eggs and lower the risk of ovarian hyperstimulation syndrome (OHSS).

2. **Embryo Transfer:** More accuracy in the embryo's placement in the uterus can double the chance of implantation thanks to methods like ultrasound-guided embryo transfer. Pregnancy rates have also been demonstrated to increase with the development of blastocyst transfer, which transfers the embryo during the 5-day stage as opposed to the customary 3-day stage.

Human Growth Hormone (HGH) and Platelet-Rich Plasma (PRP) in Enhancing Fertility:

The possibility of novel treatments like human growth hormone (HGH) and platelet-rich plasma (PRP) to improve fertility in women with problems related to the endometrial lining or low ovarian reserve is being investigated.

1. **PRP Therapy:** To promote tissue regeneration and enhance ovarian function or uterine receptivity, a patient's own platelets are concentrated and injected into the ovaries or uterus. According to preliminary research, PRP may enhance endometrial thickness and egg quality, raising the likelihood of a successful implantation for IVF recipients.

2. **HGH Therapy:** To enhance egg quality during IVF, especially in women with decreased ovarian reserve, human growth hormone is utilized as an adjuvant therapy. It is believed that HGH increases the ovaries' receptivity to stimulation, producing eggs of higher quality and possibly increasing the likelihood of pregnancy.

Although these treatments are still in the experimental phase, preliminary findings indicate that they may be useful in treating infertility.

PGT Testing and Genetic Screening in ART:

Preimplantation Genetic Testing (PGT) is a novel technique that checks embryos for genetic defects before implantation in conjunction with in vitro fertilization (IVF). Three main categories of PGT exist:

1. **PGT-A (Preimplantation Genetic Testing for Aneuploidy):** Tests for chromosomal abnormalities, like extra or missing chromosomes (e.g., Down syndrome), are performed on embryos. Choosing embryos with regular chromosomes can increase IVF success rates and lower the chance of miscarriage.

2. **PGT-M (Preimplantation Genetic Testing for Monogenic Disorders):** This test looks for certain hereditary conditions that are known to run in one or both parents, such Tay-Sachs disease or cystic fibrosis.

3. Preimplantation genetic testing for structural rearrangements, or **PGT-SR,** is a test used to identify

chromosomal rearrangements in embryos that may result in miscarriages or genetic disorders in the offspring.

By minimizing the danger of genetic diseases and increasing the likelihood of a successful pregnancy, genetic screening enables medical professionals to choose the healthiest embryos for transfer.

5.3 Financial and Ethical Aspects

Even though ART has improved many people's lives, there are still moral and financial issues that need to be taken into account.

Legal and Moral Implications of Using ART: Using ART brings up a number of legal and moral issues, especially in relation to the status of donor gametes, embryos, and surrogacy.

1. **Embryo Freezing and Disposal**: Following IVF, one ethical conundrum is what to deal with extra embryos. Should they be destroyed, given to other couples, or put to use in research? Diverse nations

and religious sects have different takes on this matter.

2. **Third-Party Reproduction:** There are intricate legal and moral issues when using surrogates, donor sperm, or eggs. Any ART agreement needs to address issues including the child's rights, parental rights, and donor anonymity.

3. **Genetic Screening:** Although preimplantation genetic testing (PGT) can lower the likelihood of genetic abnormalities being passed down, it also raises ethical questions around "designer babies" and the possibility that parents will choose embryos based on features other than medical ones, such gender or physical attributes.

ART clinics need to carefully tread these ethical waters, making sure that operations adhere to regulatory requirements and that patients are properly informed.

Expenses Associated with Fertility Treatments and Financial Planning:

ART procedures, especially IVF, can be expensive. IVF treatments can cost anywhere from $12,000 to $20,000, and many couples need more than one cycle to have a child. Medication, lab fees, and future procedures like egg retrieval or genetic testing could incur additional costs.

1. **Financial Planning:** Couples thinking about ART need to set aside money for both the initial consultations and treatments as well as continuing costs. Couples can better prepare for the financial effects of ART by creating a thorough financial strategy.

2. **Cost-Benefit Analysis:** Couples should take into account the possible emotional stress and uncertainty associated with ART, as well as the financial and emotional consequences of many treatment cycles.

Alternative Financial Support and Insurance Coverage: ART coverage varies greatly depending on the insurance company and the area. Certain drugs or diagnostic tests may be covered by some plans, while no fertility treatments may be covered at all by others. It's critical to comprehend insurance coverage and look into other sources for financial assistance.

1. **Alternative Financing Options:** Fertility clinics offer financing options that can give loans or

payment plans for assisted reproductive technologies (ART). Furthermore, couples pursuing fertility treatments can apply for grants or other financial aid from certain non-profit organizations.

Patients are urged to speak up for themselves and investigate all of their alternatives in order to increase accessibility to ART.

The development of assisted reproductive technologies (ART) has given infertile people and couples new options. This chapter has given a thorough overview of the complex field of reproductive health, covering everything from comprehending standard ART techniques to investigating the newest advancements and navigating ethical and financial concerns. ART will surely become more and more important in assisting people in realizing their aspirations of becoming parents as science and technology advance, with making wise selections being crucial to this path.

CHAPTER 6

LOSS OF PREGNANCY AND MISCARRIAGE

One of the most tragic experiences in a person's life can be miscarriage or pregnancy loss. Comprehending the intricacies associated with miscarriage is crucial for both psychological recovery and prospective family planning. This chapter seeks to offer a comprehensive examination of the reasons for miscarriages, as well as coping mechanisms for both people and families, as well as suggestions for future pregnancy planning.

6.1 Comprehending the Causes of Miscarriages

Studies indicate that between 10% and 20% of known pregnancies terminate spontaneously before the 20th week of pregnancy. Miscarriage is a common occurrence. For people who are impacted, knowing the underlying causes is crucial since it can inform decisions and actions in the future.

Typical Causes of Pregnancy Loss at an Early Age:

Most miscarriages happen in the first trimester and are frequently caused by circumstances outside of the woman's control. Typical reasons include:

1. **Chromosomal Abnormalities:** These defects in the embryo are the most common cause of miscarriage, accounting for 50–70% of cases. These can be the consequence of early cell division or faults made during fertilization, which can produce genetically unviable embryos.

2. **Implantation Problems:** Occasionally, the embryo does not properly implant in the uterine lining. This might be brought on by inadequate blood supply to the uterus or a thin endometrial lining.

3. **Hormonal Imbalances:** Early pregnancy loss can result from disorders such luteal phase deficiency, in which the body fails to produce enough progesterone to maintain pregnancy.

Genetic, Environmental, and Hormonal Risk Factors:

Miscarriage risk can be influenced by a number of risk factors, such as:

1. **Genetic Factors:** The probability of chromosomal abnormalities in embryos might be influenced by the genetic conditions of the parents. People who have balanced translocations may become pregnant again and again.

2. **Environmental Factors:** There is a connection between a higher risk of miscarriage and exposure to certain environmental pollutants, including radiation, heavy metals, and pesticides. Risk is also increased by lifestyle choices including smoking and binge drinking.

3. **Hormonal Factors**: Diseases including thyroid issues and polycystic ovarian syndrome (PCOS) can alter hormone levels, which in turn might impair the viability of a pregnancy.

Medical Disorders Associated with Miscarriage:

The following illnesses can increase the chance of miscarriage:

1. **Uterine Abnormalities:** Fibroids, polyps, and congenital malformations are examples of structural problems within the uterus that might interfere with

implantation and raise the risk of miscarriage.

2. **Autoimmune Disorders:** The body's capacity to sustain a pregnancy may be hampered by illnesses like lupus or antiphospholipid syndrome.

3. **Infections:** Sexually transmitted infections (STIs) are among the diseases that can raise the chance of miscarriage. Infections including listeria and cytomegalovirus (CMV) have also been connected to miscarriage.

Not only is it crucial for bereaved people to comprehend these causes, but it's also critical for anyone hoping to improve their health during a future pregnancy.

6.2 Recovering after Miscarriage

Each person and couple has a unique route to navigate when dealing with a miscarriage. Relationships, families, and professional resources must provide support and understanding due to the potentially severe emotional and psychological effects.

Child Support and Therapy Resources:

It is imperative that those who have suffered a miscarriage get emotional support. This could consist of:

1. **Counseling:** Seeking professional counseling or therapy can offer a secure setting for discussing emotions such as perplexity, rage, and loss. People have found that cognitive-behavioral therapy (CBT) is especially useful in processing their experiences and creating coping mechanisms.

2. **Support Groups:** Participating in a support group for women who have lost a pregnancy can help to build a sense of belonging and mutual understanding. Participants can discuss their experiences and coping mechanisms, which can be very beneficial and reassuring.

Comprehending Lament and Recovery Following Pregnancy Loss:

After a miscarriage, grief is frequently complicated and can take many different forms:

1. **Emotional Reactions:** Sadness, guilt, and worry are typical emotions. Recognizing these feelings as

legitimate components of the grieving process is crucial. Grieving is a personal experience for each individual and cannot be judged as right or wrong.

2. **Physical Symptoms:** Fatigue, changes in appetite, and trouble sleeping are just a few of the physical symptoms that can result from grief. For general wellbeing, treating these symptoms with self-care techniques or expert assistance is essential.

It's crucial that people treat themselves gently while they heal since it takes time. Celebrating tiny milestones and commemorating the pregnancy in meaningful ways might assist with the healing journey.

The Function of Family and Partner Assistance in Recovery:

A partner's and family's support can have a big influence on the recovery process:

1. **Open Communication:** Promoting candid conversations about emotions and experiences helps deepen bonds between people. As a pair, partners may choose to go through counseling to work

through their grief.

2. **Creating Rituals:** Memorials or rituals created in remembrance of a miscarried pregnancy can provide solace to bereaved families. This may be doing something symbolic, like lighting a candle or planting a tree to remember the due day.

3. **Understanding Variations in Grief:** It's important to acknowledge that different people may experience grief in various ways. empathetic that grief is a personal experience, partners may need to be empathetic and patient with them as they traverse their emotional landscapes.

Although grieving a miscarriage is a difficult path, healing and finally serenity can come with time, understanding, and support.

6.3 Making Plans for Upcoming Pregnancies

Many people and couples want to consider the possibilities of getting pregnant again after suffering a loss. It is essential to comprehend how to assess underlying problems and optimize health throughout this planning phase.

Medical Assessment Following a Miscarriage:

A medical assessment after a miscarriage can assist in determining any possible underlying problems:

1. **Follow-Up visits:** To talk about the miscarriage and any required testing, make follow-up visits with a healthcare professional. Blood tests to measure hormone levels and genetic testing for both parents to find any chromosomal abnormalities may be part of a comprehensive review.

2. **Ultrasound and Imaging**: Imaging procedures, such hysterosalpingography (HSG) or ultrasounds, might assist in identifying any uterine structural problems that might be a factor in subsequent miscarriages.

These assessments can offer insightful information and direct future conception planning.

How to Improve Your Chances of a Healthy Pregnancy:

Taking proactive measures to improve one's health can

raise the likelihood of a fruitful pregnancy:

1. **Healthy Lifestyle Choices:** Reducing alcohol and tobacco use, eating a balanced diet, and exercising frequently can all help to enhance general health and fertility. Before getting pregnant, it's also a good idea to include prenatal vitamins, especially folic acid.

2. **Stress Management**: Reducing stress through yoga, meditation, or therapy can improve the environment in which a person conceives and becomes pregnant. To become pregnant, mental health is just as important as physical health.

3. **Preconception Counseling:** Engaging in preconception counseling with a healthcare provider can assist identify potential risk factors and provide specific advice for optimizing health before attempting to conceive again.

Comprehending Recurrent Miscarriages and Their Possible Cure:

Having several miscarriages can be especially upsetting for certain people. Recurrent miscarriage, which is characterized by two or more recurrent miscarriages, calls for additional assessment:

1. **Investigating Causes:** Extensive assessments ought to delve into plausible reasons for recurrent miscarriages, including but not limited to genetic predispositions, hormone dysregulation, immunological conditions, and anomalies in the uterus. Determining these problems is essential to creating a customized therapy strategy.

2. **Potential Treatments:** Hormonal therapy, such as progesterone supplements, lifestyle changes, or surgical procedures to correct uterine anatomy, may be used to treat recurrent miscarriages. To increase the likelihood of a successful pregnancy, sophisticated reproductive methods like IVF plus PGT may be advised in specific situations.

Knowing the causes of repeat miscarriages might enable people and couples to pursue the best solutions for their particular circumstances.

Losing a pregnancy and suffering a miscarriage are deeply felt events that affect not only individuals but also families and couples. Navigating this difficult journey requires knowing the reasons behind miscarriage, creating coping mechanisms, and making plans for subsequent pregnancies. After a loss, people and couples can find hope and healing with the right support, medical evaluation, and proactive health management.

CHAPTER 7

HORMONE BALANCING NATURAL METHODS

For general health, and especially for conception, hormonal balance is essential. Hormones are important biological regulators that affect metabolism, mood, and reproductive health, among other things. This chapter analyzes the role that hormone balance plays in fertility, looks at dietary and lifestyle modifications that promote hormonal health, and looks at herbal therapies that can aid in reestablishing hormonal balance.

7.1 Hormonal Balance Is Critical for Fertility

Reproductive health depends on maintaining hormonal balance, which affects everything from ovulation to regular menstruation and overall fertility.

The Impact of Hormone Mismatches on Reproductive Health:

A number of problems with reproductive health can result from hormonal abnormalities. Key hormones involved in the reproductive cycle include estrogen, progesterone, testosterone, and thyroid hormones. An imbalance may lead to:

1. **Irregular Menstrual Cycles:** It might be difficult to conceive when there are disruptions in the hormonal signals that control the menstrual cycle, resulting in irregular or skipped periods.

2. **Ovulatory Dysfunction:** Anovulatory insufficiency, or anovulation, is a major cause of infertility and can be caused by imbalances that impact ovulation.

3. **Diseases like endometriosis and PCOS:** Fertility can be hampered by both endometriosis and polycystic ovarian syndrome (PCOS), which are both frequently associated with increased testosterone levels.

Hormonal Imbalance Signs and Symptoms:

It is essential to identify the symptoms of a hormone imbalance in order to take prompt action. Typical signs and symptoms could be:

1. **Irregular Periods:** Hormonal problems may be indicated by changes in cycle length, skipped periods, or heavy bleeding.

2. **Mood Swings:** Anxiety, despair, or irritability can result from hormone imbalances, which have a substantial impact on mood.

3. **Weight Changes:** Hormonal changes, including those involving insulin, cortisol, and thyroid hormones, may be the cause of unexplained weight gain or loss.

4. **Excessive Fatigue and Sleep Problems:** Hormonal imbalance can also be indicated by persistent exhaustion, sleeplessness, or sleep disruptions.

Standard Hormone-Associated Conditions:

Hormonal abnormalities are especially linked to the following disorders:

- **Hypothyroidism:** Symptoms like lethargy, weight gain, and irregular menstruation can result from an underactive thyroid. Reproductive health and general hormonal balance depend on healthy thyroid function.

- **Adrenal exhaustion:** The inability of the adrenal glands to produce enough cortisol causes symptoms like exhaustion, anxiety, and hormonal imbalance. Chronic stress can cause adrenal fatigue.

For those who want to achieve hormonal balance and maximize their reproductive health, understanding these components is essential.

7.2 Modifications to Diet and Lifestyle

Modifications to diet and lifestyle can have a significant effect on hormone balance, supporting general health and reproductive health.

Foods To Promote Appropriate Hormone Levels:
Hormone regulation is significantly influenced by dietary decisions. Among the food suggestions are:

1. **Healthy Fats:** By lowering inflammation and promoting brain function, including foods high in omega-3 fatty acids, such as walnuts, flaxseeds, and

fatty fish (salmon, mackerel), can help regulate hormones.

2. **Whole Foods:** A diet high in fruits, vegetables, whole grains, lean meats, and other whole foods provide vital vitamins and minerals that promote hormonal balance. Brussels sprouts, kale, and other cruciferous vegetables have substances that aid in the metabolism of excess estrogen.

3. **Fiber-Rich Foods:** Consuming more fiber helps improve gut health and help control insulin, both of which are essential for hormone balance. Vegetables, whole grains, legumes, and fruits are foods high in dietary fiber.

Minimizing Endocrine Disruptor Exposure:

Hormonal health can be greatly impacted by environmental influences. Hormone balance can be improved by lowering exposure to endocrine disruptors, or chemicals that interfere with hormone activities. Important tactics consist of:

1. **Avoiding Plastics:** Reducing the amount of plastic containers you use, particularly for food and drink,

can help lower your exposure to phthalates and bisphenol A (BPA), two chemicals that are known to disrupt hormones.

2. **Selecting Organic Produce:** Choosing organic produce helps reduce your exposure to pesticides and herbicides, which can upset your hormone balance.

3. **Natural Cleaning Products:** Using natural personal care and cleaning products will help lower exposure to man made chemicals that might have an adverse effect on hormone health.

Fitness, Stress Reduction, and Sleep Enhancement:
Hormonal balance can be greatly enhanced by including physical activity, controlling stress, and improving sleep patterns:

1. **Regular Exercise:** Physical activity on a regular basis can help manage weight, lower stress levels, and increase insulin sensitivity. Try to incorporate strength training, flexibility training, and cardiovascular activity into your routine.

2. **Stress Management:** Hormonal imbalances and

adrenal exhaustion can result from prolonged, high levels of stress. Stress reduction methods include deep breathing exercises, yoga, and mindfulness meditation.

3. **Sleep Hygiene:** Ensuring adequate sleep is crucial for controlling hormones. Enhancing sleep quality can be achieved by establishing a regular sleep pattern, coming up with a relaxing night time ritual, and making sure the sleep environment is comfortable.

A better hormonal environment can be fostered by people adopting certain dietary and lifestyle adjustments, which is especially advantageous for reproductive health.

7.3 All-Natural Hormone Balance Treatments

Natural therapies can supplement dietary and lifestyle modifications by providing extra assistance for hormone balancing.

Herbal Supplements and Their Function in Hormone Regulation:

Traditional uses of a few herbal remedies to promote hormonal health include:

1. **Maca Root:** Known for its adaptogenic qualities, maca root may support the adrenal glands, which in turn may help control hormone levels and enhance fertility.

2. Vitex (Chaste Tree Berry): Studies have indicated that vitex can help balance the levels of progesterone and estrogen, which helps to control menstrual cycles and reduce PMS symptoms.

3. **Ashwagandha:** This adaptogen is a helpful supplement for hormonal balance because it supports thyroid function and helps fight stress.

To guarantee safety and effectiveness, it is imperative to speak with a healthcare professional before beginning any herbal supplementation.

Yoga, Acupuncture, and Mindfulness Exercises:
Complementary therapies can also play a key role in promoting hormonal balance:

1. **Acupuncture:** This method of traditional Chinese medicine may help promote hormonal balance by enhancing blood flow to the reproductive organs, regulating the menstrual cycle, and reducing stress.

2. **Yoga:** Certain yoga postures can improve flexibility and lower stress levels, which supports hormonal balance in general. Practices that emphasize deep breathing and relaxation are particularly useful for regulating cortisol levels.

3. **Mindfulness Practices:** Stress and anxiety reduction are essential for preserving hormonal balance. Mindfulness practices like meditation and deep breathing can help.

Replacement Therapy with Bioidentical Hormones: When It's Right:

For certain people, bioidentical hormone replacement therapy (BHRT) could be a good choice, especially if they are dealing with severe hormonal abnormalities brought on by menopause or other conditions:

1. **Understanding BHRT:** Bioidentical hormones are used to correct hormone imbalances or deficiencies

because they are chemically identical to those produced by the human body.

2. **Indications for Use:** Those with severe hormonal imbalances that impair quality of life, such as menopause symptoms, low testosterone in men, or hormonal imbalances in women with PCOS, may benefit from BHRT.

3. **Speaking with an Expert:** Working with a licensed healthcare professional is crucial to figuring out whether BHRT is the right course of action, as well as to track the efficacy of the treatment and any possible adverse effects.

Natural therapies can help people take charge of their hormonal health and promote fertility in addition to food and lifestyle modifications.

To achieve the best possible health and fertility, hormonal balance must be achieved. Overall well-being can be greatly impacted by realizing the significance of hormone balance, implementing educated food and lifestyle adjustments, and investigating alternative therapies. People who want to balance their hormones should address the problem holistically, taking into account all facets of their health and obtaining medical advice as needed. They can achieve this by establishing a more hormonally balanced environment that supports both general vigor and reproductive health.

CHAPTER 8

CONSERVING FUTURE FERTILITY

Understanding the complexities of fertility and its preservation becomes increasingly important as people negotiate their life and career aspirations. Natural changes occur in fertility throughout life, especially in women. Fertility is not continuous. This chapter covers many methods for preserving fertility, gives a thorough explanation of how fertility decreases with age, and highlights lifestyle decisions that might support long-term reproductive health.

8.1 Comprehending the Decline in Fertility with Age

A dynamic component of human health, fertility is susceptible to variations brought on by biological, environmental, and behavioral variables.

How Fertility Affects Ages Between 20 and 40: Women's

fertility gradually declines starting in their late 20s, peaking in their late teens to early 20s. Fertility begins to diminish at the age of 30, and by the late thirties, the decline is accelerating. This downturn may appear as:

1. **More Difficulty Conceiving:** As women age, their chances of conceiving decline, with women in their 40s experiencing particularly difficult times.

2. **Higher chance of Miscarriage:** Because of chromosomal abnormalities in eggs, older age is linked to a higher chance of miscarriage.

- Age-related factors can still affect reproductive health in males, even though fertility can be reasonably constant into their 40s and beyond. These considerations include:

  - **Sperm Quality:** Sperm motility, morphology, and general quality may deteriorate with age in males, which may have an effect on fertility.

The Reasons Behind Declining Egg Quality Over Time: Fertility is heavily dependent on egg quality, which is declining due to a number of factors:

1. **Natural Attrition:** Due to natural processes, a woman's egg supply is limited at birth and gradually decreases. A woman may lose a sizable portion of her eggs by the time she is in her 30s.

2. **Disorders of the Chromosome:** The probability of chromosomal abnormalities in eggs rises with age in women, and this might result in genetic diseases or sterility in the progeny.

The Effect of Postponing Parenthood on Fertility: Delaying having children has become more and more frequent as a result of cultural and individual influences, such as desires for education and profession. Nonetheless, there may be important consequences for fertility from this delay:

1. **Age-Related Infertility:** Due to decreased egg quality and quantity, couples who try to conceive later may have more difficulties.

2. **Increased Medical Intervention:** Success rates with assisted reproductive technologies (ART) may be lower in persons who postpone conceiving compared to younger individuals.

Anyone hoping to maintain their fertility and contemplating future family planning must be aware of these variables.

8.2 Options for Preserving Fertility

The number of choices for maintaining reproductive capacity increases along with awareness of the reduction in fertility. There are numerous ways to support individuals and couples in securing their future fertility.

Egg Freezing: Procedure, Costs, and Success Rates: Women can freeze their eggs, a process known as oocyte cryopreservation, to preserve them for later use. Usually, the procedure entails:

1. **Ovarian Stimulation:** The ovaries are stimulated to generate numerous eggs through the administration of hormonal medicines.

2. **Egg Retrieval:** After they reach maturity, a small surgical incision is made to remove the eggs.

3. **Freezing:** Cryopreservation methods are employed to freeze the recovered eggs.

Success Rates: The age of the woman during egg retrieval and the quantity of frozen eggs are major factors in the success of egg freezing. Generally speaking: - When thawed and utilized for IVF later, eggs frozen before the age of 35 have the highest success rates.

- The person's overall health and reproductive history also have an impact on success rates.

Costs: Depending on the region and clinic, egg freezing might have a considerable cost variation. Important cost factors consist of:

1. **Starting Charges:** usually, without including the expense of medication, which can add a further $3,000 to $5,000, ranging from $6,000 to $15,000.

2. **Storage Fees:** There may be a $500–$1,000 annual storage charge for frozen eggs.

Freezing of Embryos for Potential Pregnancies: Another useful technique for maintaining fertility is embryo freezing, especially for IVF couples. This technique involves:

1. **Fertilization:** To make embryos, eggs are taken out and fertilized in a lab using sperm.

2. **Freezing:** After viability, embryos are preserved for later use.

Benefits of Embryo Freezing:

1. Greater success rates in comparison to frozen eggs since the quality of the embryos is evaluated before freezing.

2. Because pre-frozen embryos can be thawed and implanted without the need for ovarian stimulation, it makes future IVF rounds easier and possibly less expensive.

Preservation of Ovarian Tissue and Experimental Techniques: An new method involves preserving ovarian tissue, especially for women undergoing medical treatments (such as chemotherapy) that may reduce their ability to conceive. The process includes:

1. **Surgical Removal:** To prepare it for a future transplant, a tiny amount of ovarian tissue is surgically removed.

2. **Experimental Status:** This method is still primarily experimental but has shown potential in specific circumstances.

Other Experimental Techniques: Research is being conducted on methods like ovarian rejuvenation and stem cell utilization, which may provide future opportunities for fertility preservation and restoration.

Examining these possibilities can enable people to make knowledgeable decisions about their reproductive futures.

8.3 Lifestyle Decisions for the Long-Term Health of Fertility

Lifestyle decisions are crucial to preserving reproductive health, even while medical procedures can help preserve fertility.

Practices That Encourage Longevity in Fertility: A few lifestyle choices can improve fertility over the long run, such as:

1. **Avoiding Excessive Alcohol and Smoking:** Smoking and excessive alcohol use can both have a deleterious effect on the quality of eggs and sperm and are associated with lower fertility.

2. **Managing Weight:** Hormonal balance depends on maintaining a healthy weight. Both being underweight and being obese can interfere with ovulation and menstrual periods, as well as cause illnesses like PCOS.

Controlling Stress and Its Impact on Unborn Children: Hormonal balance and reproductive health can be significantly impacted by prolonged stress. Among the techniques for managing stress are:

1. **Mindfulness and Relaxation Techniques:** Deep breathing exercises, yoga, and meditation are among the practices that can assist lower stress levels.

2. **Physical Activity:** Frequent exercise helps support hormonal balance and enhance general health by acting as an efficient stress reliever.

The Significance of a Balanced Diet and Regular Exercise in Sustaining Fertility: In order to maintain fertility, diet and exercise are essential:

1. **Balanced Diet:** Essential nutrients that support reproductive health can be obtained from a diet high in whole foods, such as fruits, vegetables, lean

meats, and healthy fats.

2. **Regular Exercise:** Maintaining a healthy weight, enhancing circulation, and lowering stress are all benefits that accrue to fertility when one engages in regular, moderate exercise.

A person's chances of conceiving a child successfully in the future can be greatly increased by incorporating certain lifestyle habits.

Understanding the normal reduction in reproductive capacity, looking into fertility preservation alternatives, and embracing a healthy lifestyle are all necessary to preserve fertility for the future. By being proactive and aware about these elements, individuals can take substantial measures toward maintaining their fertility, ensuring that they are equipped for family planning when the time is right. To receive individualized advice and to stay up to date on the most recent advancements in reproductive health and fertility preservation methods, it is imperative to speak with medical professionals.

CHAPTER 9

EXCEPTIONAL HEMORRHAGES AND THEIR REASONS

For many people, unusual bleeding can be a serious worry that has to be addressed because it frequently points to underlying health problems. The objectives of this chapter are to clarify the distinctions between abnormal and normal bleeding, investigate the causes and management options for abnormal uterine bleeding, and talk about the effects of abnormal bleeding on fertility. Comprehending these facets is crucial for efficacious diagnosis and treatment.

9.1 Typical versus Atypical Hemorrhage

It is essential to distinguish between normal and abnormal bleeding in order to identify any health problems.

Comprehending Typical Menstrual Patterns: Bleeding typically lasts two to seven days throughout a menstrual cycle that lasts 21 to 35 days. Typical menstruation is typified by:

1. **Flow:** Because of the modest menstrual flow, sanitary goods must be used consistently.

2. **Coherence**: Blood can contain tiny clots and range in color from bright red to dark brown.

3. **Symptom Formation:** Although some people may feel pain or cramps, the symptoms shouldn't be incapacitating.

Typical Reasons for Unexplained Bleeding: Any bleeding that takes place outside of the regular menstrual cycle is referred to as abnormal uterine bleeding (AUB). Typical reasons include:

1. **Fibroids:** Noncancerous growths in the uterus that can lead to pelvic pain, heavy menstrual flow, and extended periods.

2. **Polyps:** Benign, microscopic growths affixed to the uterine wall that may also be a factor in irregular pattern bleeding.

3. **Hormonal Imbalances:** Variations in progesterone and estrogen levels can cause irregular bleeding. These variations are frequently observed in perimenopause or in disorders like polycystic

ovarian syndrome (PCOS).

Diagnosis using Hysteroscopy, Biopsies, and Ultrasounds: AUB's fundamental causes must be accurately diagnosed in order to begin a successful treatment plan. Typical diagnostic techniques consist of:

1. **Ultrasounds:** Abdominal or transvaginal ultrasounds can be used to see within the uterus and find anomalies like polyps or fibroids.

2. **Endometrial Biopsy**: To check for anomalies, such as hyperplasia or cancer, a little sample of the uterine lining is removed.

3. **Hysteroscopy:** A minimally invasive technique that makes the uterine cavity directly visible, facilitating the identification and management of any anomalies found.

Anyone experiencing unusual bleeding must comprehend these distinctions and the diagnostic procedures involved.

9.2 Abnormal Uterine Bleeding Treatment

Options for treatment can be investigated once the

underlying cause of irregular bleeding has been determined.

Medical Treatments:

1. Abnormal uterine bleeding can be effectively managed with a number of medical interventions:

2. **Hormonal Therapy**: By stabilizing hormone levels, birth control tablets, patches, or hormonal IUDs can help control menstrual cycles and lessen severe bleeding.

3. **Non-Steroidal Anti-Inflammatory Drugs (NSAIDs):** By lowering inflammation and prostaglandin synthesis, drugs like ibuprofen help lessen pain and bleeding.

4. **Tranexamic Acid**: By encouraging blood coagulation, this antifibrinolytic drug lessens severe menstrual bleeding.

Surgical Procedures:

1. Surgical options may be taken into consideration in situations where medicinal therapy is ineffective:

2. **Dilation and Curettage (D&C)**: This treatment, which is frequently used to identify or manage

irregular bleeding, entails scraping the uterine lining to remove tissue.

3. **Endometrial Ablation:** Suitable for those who do not intend to conceive, this minimally invasive technique removes the endometrial lining to lessen or halt bleeding.

4. **Myomectomy:** Suitable for women who want to retain their fertility, this procedure removes fibroids surgically while leaving the uterus intact.

Natural Solutions: Many people look for alternative therapies to control irregular bleeding. Among the organic methods are:

1. **Dietary Adjustments**: Including iron, vitamin K, and omega-3 fatty acids in your diet can help maintain general reproductive health.

2. **Herbs:** Medicinal plants like ginger and turmeric have anti-inflammatory and menstrual-healthy properties. But prior to beginning any herbal regimen, it is imperative that you speak with a healthcare professional.

3. **Stress Reduction Techniques:** Activities like yoga, meditation, and mindfulness can help to promote

relaxation and hormonal stability, as stress can exacerbate hormone abnormalities.

The underlying cause, the degree of symptoms, and the patient's goals for reproduction all influence the therapy option.

9.3 Unusual Bleeding's Effect on Fertility

The effects of unusual bleeding on fertility and general reproductive health can be profound.

The Impact of Irregular Bleeding on Ovulation and Conception: The likelihood of conception may be impacted by irregular ovulation caused by abnormal uterine bleeding. As an illustration:

1. **Anovulation**: It might be challenging to conceive when ovulation fails to occur due to irregular menstrual cycles.

2. **Timing Interference:** Variable bleeding might make it difficult to schedule sexual activity or fertility treatments, which can make conception more difficult.

Identifying and Handling Ovulation Issues: Additional assessment is necessary if irregular ovulation coexists with abnormal bleeding. This could consist of:

1. **Hormonal Testing:** Blood tests can measure hormone levels to find out whether ovulation is taking place and to spot any irregularities in hormone levels.

2. **Treatment Options:** In cases of ovulatory dysfunction, medications such gonadotropins or clomiphene citrate can induce ovulation.

Planning for Fertility with Non-Regular Cycles: People who have irregular menstrual periods should collaborate closely with medical professionals to create a reproductive plan that takes into account their particular situation. Important tactics could be:

1. **Tracking Cycles:** Documenting menstrual cycles and accompanying symptoms in great detail can reveal patterns and support fertility planning.

2. **Medications for Fertility:** To increase the likelihood of conception, assisted reproductive technologies (ART) like in vitro fertilization (IVF)

may be advised in specific situations.

For those who are intending to become pregnant, understanding the connection between irregular bleeding and fertility is crucial in order to make educated choices and implement the necessary actions.

Unusual bleeding may be a sign of a number of underlying medical conditions, requiring thorough assessment and treatment. For those with these symptoms, it's important to know the difference between normal and abnormal bleeding, look into treatment options, and consider the effect on fertility. People can take charge of their reproductive health by being proactive and knowledgeable, which will improve their chances of achieving family planning goals and general well-being. Regular consultations with healthcare specialists can provide individualized direction and assistance, ensuring that individuals navigate these challenges efficiently.

CHAPTER 10

LGBTQ+ AND SINGLE PARENTS' FERTILITY

For single parents and LGBTQ+ couples, the path to motherhood can bring special opportunities and challenges. Parenting is a very personal experience for individuals and couples. This chapter seeks to offer a thorough examination of the family-building alternatives accessible to LGBTQ+ people and single parents, as well as the complexities involved in navigating reproductive procedures and the significance of psychological and emotional support during the process.

10.1 Choices for Family Building

LGBTQ+ people and single parents have several alternatives to consider when thinking about starting a family.

ART Choices and Fertility Monitoring for Same-Sex

Couples and Single Parents: Understanding one's reproductive health and making plans for pregnancy depend heavily on fertility tracking. Choices consist of:

1. **Cycle Monitoring:** Monitoring menstrual cycles, ovulation windows, and fertile days with apps and ovulation kits might increase the likelihood of pregnancy.

2. **Assisted Reproductive Technology (ART):** Methods including in vitro fertilization (IVF) and intrauterine insemination (IUI) can be used. For lesbian couples, these techniques might involve sperm donors; for gay male couples, they might entail single parents or egg donors.

Processes for Sperm Donation, Egg Donation, and Surrogacy: Using donor gametes or surrogacy can involve intricate procedures that call for advance planning:

Sperm Donation: Through sperm banks, individuals or couples can select anonymous or known donors, such as friends or relatives. Among the crucial factors are:

1. **Legal Agreements:** When employing known donors, it is extremely important to establish detailed legal agreements regarding parental rights and

obligations.

2. **Screening:** To guarantee donor compatibility, sperm banks normally conduct thorough health tests, which may include genetic testing.

Egg Donation: Whether via friends, relatives, or egg donor organizations, finding a suitable donor is crucial for individuals in need of eggs. Crucial actions consist of:

1. **Legal Contracts:** Clearly defined contracts that specify parental rights and obligations are necessary, just like with sperm donation.

2. **Health Assessments:** To determine their appropriateness and overall health, donors undergo medical assessments.

Surrogacy: This is a possibility for couples who are unable to conceive. Important things to think about are:

1. **Traditional vs. Gestational Surrogacy:** In traditional surrogacy, the surrogate uses her own eggs, whereas in gestational surrogacy, an embryo made with the intended parents' or donors' eggs and sperm is implanted.

2. **Legal Framework:** Surrogacy regulations differ greatly by location, demanding legal counsel to manage contracts, parental rights, and compensation.

Legal Aspects for LGBTQ+ Families in Various Countries: The legal environment that affects LGBTQ+ families differs greatly between nations and areas, which affects the family-building alternatives available:

1. **Parenting Rights:** While some jurisdictions grant a same-sex couple complete parental rights, others may need further legal action to formally establish these rights.

2. **Adoption Laws:** While adoption laws vary in terms of who can adopt and how, many jurisdictions let same-sex couples to adopt.

3. **Protection Against Discrimination:** Adoption and fertility services may be impacted by legal safeguards against discrimination based on gender identity or sexual orientation, which can vary.

It takes careful study and frequent expert advice to navigate these possibilities so that individuals and couples can make decisions that are in line with their family goals.

10.2 Getting Around Fertility Therapies

Navigating fertility treatments for LGBTQ+ people and single parents requires knowing what options are available and selecting the one that best suits their particular situation.

IUI, ICI, and IVF Customized for LGBTQ+ Pairs: The demands of LGBTQ+ couples can be catered for using a variety of fertility treatments:

1. **Intrauterine Insemination (IUI):** A popular method for single parents or lesbian couples, IUI involves injecting sperm directly into the uterus during ovulation to maximize the likelihood of conception.

2. **Intracervical Insemination (ICI):** Consists of implantation of sperm into the cervix; comparable to IUI. It might be a good choice for people who are using known donors.

3. **In Vitro Fertilization (IVF):** IVF gives same-sex male couples flexibility by enabling the generation of embryos outside of the body through the use of an

egg donor and gestational surrogate.

Adoption and Foster Care as Alternative Paths to Parenthood:

1. For LGBTQ+ people and single parents, adoption and foster care are viable routes to parenthood.

Adoption: Although the procedure differs by state, LGBTQ+ couples are becoming more and more accepted as acceptable parents. Crucial actions consist of:

1. **Selecting the Adoption Type:** There are three types of adoption: foster care, international, and domestic, each with specific needs and procedures.

2. **Legal Considerations:** Determining legal rights is essential, particularly in areas where adoptive parents who identify as LGBTQ+ are not always accepted.

Foster Care: Becoming a foster parent can be a rewarding experience. Crucial elements to take into account are as follows:

1. **Licensing Process:** To become foster parents, individuals and couples must fulfill certain requirements and go through a licensing procedure.

2. **Support Services:** Foster parents must have access

to resources and support services in order to give children a stable home.

Managing Gender Dysphoria Throughout Pregnancy: Gender dysphoria is a serious worry for transgender or non-binary people who want to get pregnant:

1. **Mental Health Support:** Getting mental health support throughout pregnancy can help with anxiety and distress associated with physical changes.

2. **Healthcare Provider Communication:** A supportive pregnancy experience can be facilitated by having open discussions on gender identity and special needs with healthcare providers.

3. **Postpartum Considerations:** Making plans for postpartum care, such as accessing mental health services and LGBTQ+ parent-focused support groups, can improve general wellbeing.

Individuals and couples can make decisions that are in line with their needs and aspirations by being aware of the subtleties surrounding various fertility treatments and routes to parenthood.

10.3 Psychological and Emotional Assistance

Being a parent can be an extremely taxing experience, and getting the correct support is essential to getting through it.

Overcoming the Emotional Difficulties of Family-Building:

When attempting to have a family, individuals and couples may encounter a variety of emotional difficulties, such as:

1. **Grief and Loss:** Dealing with losses, such ineffective fertility treatments or unsuccessful adoptions, may be part of the process, necessitating time for grieving.

2. **worry and Anxiety:** There can be a great deal of worry and anxiety associated with the unknowns surrounding fertility treatments and the difficulties involved in navigating legal systems.

Navigating Societal and Family Expectations:

1. LGBTQ+ people and single parents may face extra pressure as a result of societal and family expectations.

2. **Acceptance:** Seeking approval from loved ones and

the larger community may be very emotionally taxing, particularly in less accepting settings.

3. **Cultural Norms:** People who want to challenge conventional ideas of family may need to set boundaries and be transparent about their intentions.

Identifying Professional Counselors and Supportive Communities:

Making connections with counselors and supportive communities can significantly improve mental health during this journey:

1. **Support Groups:** Participating in groups designed just for LGBTQ+ parents or people in general can offer a secure setting for exchanging experiences, difficulties, and triumphs.

2. **Professional Counseling:** During the family-building process, seeking the assistance of mental health specialists who are knowledgeable about LGBTQ+ problems can provide tailored coping mechanisms and emotional support.

3. **Online Resources:** Forums and online platforms can help link you with people going through similar things so you can share advice and support.

In order to successfully navigate the emotional terrain of starting a family, proactive measures to find support and develop resilience are needed.

Solo parents and LGBTQ+ people face different chances and challenges on their path to parenthood. People can take charge of their own family-building by being aware of their options, managing the difficulties associated with reproductive treatments, and placing a high value on psychological and emotional support. Sustained promotion of fair access to family-building materials and reproductive services is necessary to guarantee that everyone, irrespective of sexual orientation or parental status, can fulfill their aspirations of becoming parents. LGBTQ+ people who are also single parents can successfully traverse this rewarding road toward family formation with the help of information, resiliency, and community support.

ABOUT THE AUTHOR

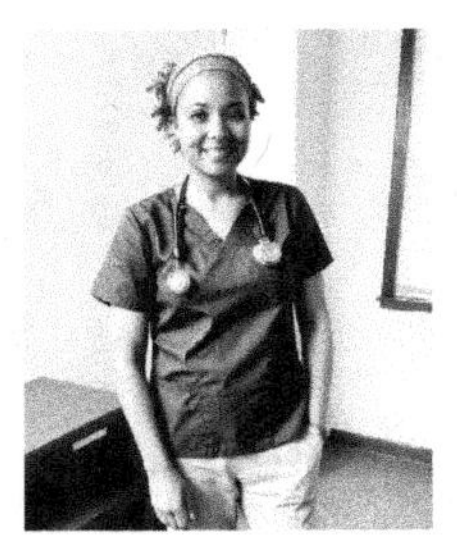 Harmony Royce is a dedicated healthcare worker who has a strong interest in holistic wellness. Harmony's extensive history in various aspects of health and wellness provides her with a wealth of knowledge and expertise that she can utilize in her writing and professional endeavors.

Harmony is a talented author who crafts thought-provoking books that inspire readers to have well-rounded, balanced lives. She writes about a variety of health-related topics, such as diet, exercise, mental health, and mindfulness. Her approachable writing style combines practical guidance with evidence-based research to make complex health concepts approachable and engaging for readers of all ages.

Harmony actively promotes the benefits of holistic health through writing, community workshops, and internet forums. Her mission is to educate and inspire people about the transformative power of self-care and healthy lifestyle choices.